YOUR KNOWLEDGE HAS VALUE

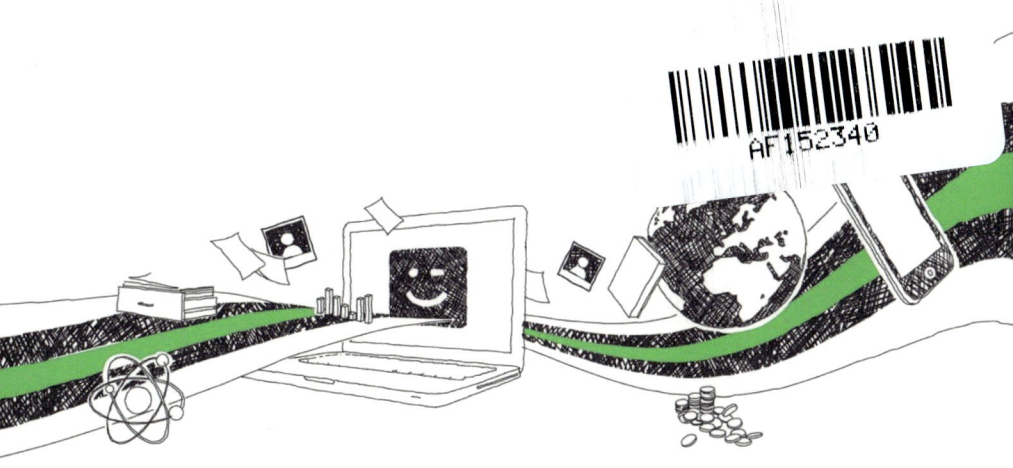

- We will publish your bachelor's and
  master's thesis, essays and papers

- Your own eBook and book -
  sold worldwide in all relevant shops

- Earn money with each sale

Upload your text at www.GRIN.com
and publish for free

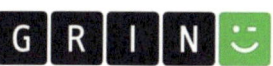

Sarah Pinsdorf

Consolidation of hospitals

Decreasing costs and increasing quality?

GRIN Verlag

Bibliografische Information der Deutschen Nationalbibliothek:

Die Deutsche Bibliothek verzeichnet diese Publikation in der Deutschen National-
bibliografie; detaillierte bibliografische Daten sind im Internet über http://dnb.d-
nb.de/ abrufbar.

Imprint:

Copyright © 2011 GRIN Verlag GmbH
Druck und Bindung: Books on Demand GmbH, Norderstedt Germany
ISBN: 978-3-656-61612-2

This book at GRIN:

http://www.grin.com/en/e-book/270276/consolidation-of-hospitals

GRIN - Your knowledge has value

Der GRIN Verlag publiziert seit 1998 wissenschaftliche Arbeiten von Studenten, Hochschullehrern und anderen Akademikern als eBook und gedrucktes Buch. Die Verlagswebsite www.grin.com ist die ideale Plattform zur Veröffentlichung von Hausarbeiten, Abschlussarbeiten, wissenschaftlichen Aufsätzen, Dissertationen und Fachbüchern.

Visit us on the internet:

http://www.grin.com/

http://www.facebook.com/grincom

http://www.twitter.com/grin_com

University of Applied Sciences Fresenius
Faculty of Economics & Media
Field of Study: Health Economics

Consolidation of Hospitals –
Decreasing costs and increasing quality?

Module SP 1.2: English – Business Acumen
Partial Module: Academic and Business Writing SS 2011

By
Sarah Pinsdorf

Due Date: 1st August 2011

Contents

Chapter 1
Introduction

Increasing cost pressure, shortage of staff, investment backlog – more and more hospitals need to merge with others to survive. Apart from the decreasing capital investments of the federal states, especially the implementation of DRGs (Monopolkommission 2008, 313) and the possibility of integrated health care lead to an enormous cost pressure.

In Germany, there is a dual hospital funding. The costs of operation are beared by payments of health insurance funds. Investment costs for new buildings or the replacement of capital goods are payed by the federal states. However, these allowances of investment are on the decrease for years, which leads to investment backlogs in hospital (Augurzky et al. 2009, 93). This implies that hospitals are supposed to invest, but their funds are too small to do so. In the long run, the economic efficiency suffers because it cannot compete with other hospitals regarding the technological progress (Augurzky et al. 2009, 13). The introduction of DRGs [*Diagnosis Related Groups*], the basis of calculation for hospitals, lead to an increasing pressure of working economically. In the old system, every day of a patient's stay in the hospital was refunded based on same-day hospital and nursing charges. In the new system, only occupant days within a predetermined period of hospitalization. The preterm discharge or a discharge exceeding the period of hospitalization results in discounts in payments, which often do not allow cost recovery (Eveslage 2006, 37-39). Accordingly, hospitals are under pressure to treat their patients fast and discharge them within the preset period. This requires efficient and economical operations. An additional burden is the growing competition in the sector of ambulatory care. As a result of the strong medical progress, more and more operations, which were formerly bound to be performed in hospital, can nowadays be done ambulant. Another innovation in the German health care system are medical service centers [*Medizinische Versorgungszentren*]. They will soon be capable to take over the primary health care in rural areas and replace major hospitals there, because they are able to work more economic (Augurzky et al. 2009, 162). On the whole, the pressure on hospitals increased steadily in the past years. Many hospitals are not capable to assert themselves on the market under today's conditions solitary. 12 per cent of the economically weak hospitals are expected to shut down by 2020. (Augurzky et al. 2009, 124). This is, apart from the already mentioned reasons, a consequence of increasing overcapacities. Many hospitals try to consolidate in order to avoid a closure. These attempts often fail, but if they are successful, a consolidation leads to decreasing costs and increasing quality. In the following paper, there is a general consideration of consolidation conditions and possibilities and especially a close look at the advantages and disadvantages of consolidations regarding cost savings and quality improvement.

Chapter 2
Consolidation in general

Consolidation can be defined as the "Combining [of] two or more firms through purchase, merger, or ownership transfer to form a new firm" (Business Dictionary, 2011). In addition to all rights, assets and debts are also transferred to the newly merged venture (Greulich 2005, 108). The development of a consolidation averages one year from the first concrete idea to the signing of a contract (Steffen and Offermanns 2011, 4). The entire integration takes one to three years on average (Steffen and Offermanns 2011, 6).

Aims

The principal aim of many consolidations is the achievement of an economical size of the company. (Steffen and Offermanns 2011, 4).
Additional aims are primarily limited to the divisions market, resources and costs. The secondary aims market expansion, quality intensification and the control of the patients' flow are to improve the competitive situation at the market. Common use of resources, increased productivity and profitability as well as the exchange of experiences and quality intensification shall lead to an improved access to resources. The aim of decreased personal and material costs can be reached through the downsizing of infrastructure, staff savings, reorganisation of processes and the elimination of constructional problems (Rippmann, 5-7).

Fusion stages

According to Konrad Rippmann the process of consolidation can be divided into four phases (2007, 11-17). The preliminary decision takes three months on average. In the first instance, the decision of general principle is made. There are two possibilities: two companies merge and form a new company or one company buys another one out. In the following step, the positioning, a valuation of the own business culture is worked out. Besides the actual culture, there is also a desired value of how the culture should be. The criteria for the business culture are innovation and the readiness to assume a risk, customer orientation, costs orientation, preciseness and classification, focus on results, autonomy of employees, team orientation and the willingness to cooperate with other companies. Afterwards, the consolidation partner is examined through a well-structured battery of questions, which is divided into four category groups with three questions each.

The four categories are cooperation, own job profile, external job profile and intrinsic motivation. In the first category cooperation the stumbling blocks of cooperation, the general goals and the specific goals are identified. The own job profile contains three questions: 1. What do I like to do? 2. What am I good at? 3. What do others cherish me for? The third category external job profile deals with the questions 'What does Mr. X like to do?', 'What is Mr. X good at?' and 'What do I appreciate about Mr. X?'. The endmost category intrinsic motivation differentiates between 'one third I enjoy to do', 'one third I accept' and 'one third I am glad to hand over'.

Thereafter, a framework is developed which is communicated at an early stage to the public. In the second phase, the consolidation, agreements of guidelines and framework requirements are made and measures and aims are exactly defined. Furthermore, the preliminary consolidated area of responsibility is set and the employees are instructed and qualified. In this stage, the conceptual framework is completed. In the realization phase, all fundamental practice-related steps are finalized. This includes the formation of an internal supervision team, the adoption of a human resources management, detection of data and the implementation of the strategy. The fourth phase is about optimization of processes. First, the actual status is captured. Then, it is examined if the stadium of the project work is completed and if the company organisation structure is established. As long as the requirements are fulfilled, the company turns back to its day-to-day business. During further progress of the optimization, rearrangements are communicated internal and external. The development of new business areas and products can be started.

Types of consolidation

There are three different types of consolidation: the horizontal, the vertical and the conglomerate consolidation. The horizontal consolidation deals with the merger of two companies which are on the same level of provision of services (Horzella 2010, 28). The consolidation partners can be hospitals and groups of clinics, but also health insurances. In the vertical consolidation, companies of different levels of provision of services merge to a new unit (Horzella 2010, 28). This can be the merger of a regular hospital for acute cases and a rehab hospital. Another example is the merger of an ambulant service provider and a hospital. The conglomerate consolidation takes place between companies of different branches of trade and of different levels of production and service. The aim is to open up new business portfolio (Horzella 2010, 28). An example for this case is the merger of a manufacturer of medical devices and a hospital service.

Legal criteria

Hospital mergers are, like all other business combinations, subject to the Federal Cartel Office's merger control (§§ 35 ff. GWB). Merger controls are subdivided into formal and material merger controls (Müller-Groh 2002, 32). Whereas the formal merger control deals with the application areas (§§ 35, 36 Abs. 2, 37 GWB) and the execution (§§ 40 ff. GWB), the material merger control focusses on the permission and prohibition of consolidations (§§ 36 Abs. 1, 42 GWB). Not all hospital consolidations have to bear merger controls, but only the consolidations, whose partners reached worldwide more than 500 million Euro (§35 GWB) in the last business year before the consolidation. In the inland, it is determined that at least one of the involved companies should make more than 25 million Euro sales proceeds, another one should have made more than 5 million Euro (§ 35 GWB). As a consequence, many hospitals in Germany are not subjected to merger controls. Only consolidations with the participation of big private hospital chains or university clinics are of economical importance and are therefore controlled by the Federal Cartel Office (Monopolkommission 2008, 317). Hospital mergers with no relevance for the Federal Cartel Office are nevertheless in the majority of cases checked by the hospital and planning authority (Steffen and Offermanns 2011, 4).

Chapter 3
Advantages of Consolidation of Hospitals

A consolidation of hospitals leads to synergy effects which are useful for the cooperating partners. These synergetic effects can be divided into operative effects, effects on the production management, fiscal effects, administrative effects and also in effects on the research and the development. The hospital gains great potential concerning cost-cutting measures, if these synergies are carried out (Köninger 2008, 122). The operative synergy is about the merging of the same functions. This leads to savings of production factors because, for example, expensive equipment does not have to be bought twice (Klauber, Rober and Schnellschmidt 2006, 60). Altogether, the operative synergetic effects lead to decreasing general expenses and to an increasing economic efficiency (Budzinski and Kerber 2003, 42). A better device usage and an internal division of work with specialization advantages are the achievement of synergies in production management. The higher number of patients accompanied by the increased material usage offer the implementation of decreased purchase prices (Budzinski and Kerber 2003, 43). Furthermore, the central stock and reserve holdings can be optimized because instead of many small warehouses there is now one big central warehouse. Consumable materials and unusual medicines do not have have to be in stock twice. Fiscal synergies strengthen the bargaining position towards banks concerning capital stock condition (Budzinski and Kerber 2003, 43). The banks' willingness to invest grows with the size of the requesting company. The administrative synergies can lead to higher administration and management skills. This is often the case, when a company has to merge because of its bad economic position, following the doings of an unqualified management (Budzinski and Kerber 2003, 43). A better realization of technological and financial intensive innovations is often the result of research and development synergies. These synergetic effects are especially important when it comes to the market launch of products with high development costs. As a result of the extensive regulations on test series, the launch of medical devices and medicines takes a long time and is cost-intensive (Budzinsiki and Kerber 2003, 43-44). Small hospitals with little capital resources often cannot afford these market launches and therefore have competitive disadvantages.

Apart from the different synergetic effects, there are other advantages of consolidation which are useful for hospitals. The buyout or the consolidation with another hospital leads to a lower competition on patients (Budzinski and Kerber 2003, 52). This is an advantage for both participating hospitals. They do not have to compete against each other but can share their patients and profits.

In addition, positive economies of scale can be achieved, which are a result of the growing production output. The synergy of production management leads to cost savings. These advantages are especially useful at horizontal consolidations but only if it comes to the integration of business parts (Budzinski and Kerber 2003, 64-65). They are not adjuvant, if there is an integration only on the enterprise level (Klauber, Robra and Schnellschmidt 2007, 60).

Further advantages come up through the formation of hospital chains. Marketing advantages, which convey high quality standard and outstanding services to the customer, can be realised (Monopolkommission 2008, 316).

Estimated or expected reductions of costs are often overvalued and therefore not reached. There is a high probability of achieving estimated cost reductions, if the company works out a detailed strategy for the performance structure right at the beginning of the restructuring process. A fast implementation of the new strategy helps to end inefficient operations immediately (Vetter and Hoffmann 2005, 80).

Chapter 4
Disadvantages of Consolidation of Hospitals

In a study of the Deutsches Krankenhausinstitut (DKI), it could be proved that many consolidations fail. The reasons for the failures are diverse, but often based on insufficient preparation, poor information and integration of employees as well as inadequate implementation of integration measures (Steffen and Offermanns 2011, 3). Furthermore, personal, planning and organisational reasons play an important role (Steffen and Offermanns 2011, 4). Whereas hard factors, like financial situation, property relations and hospital planning, are in the majority of cases sufficiently checked, the soft factors, like organisational and strategical aspects, personnel costs, personnel development measures or legal relationships, are often disregarded (Steffen and Offermanns 2011, 5). This can lead to problems in the further course of the consolidation process or even to the failure of the consolidation.

Problematical are high horizontal integrations of enterprises because they lead to a decline of innovation activity and variety of products (Budzinski and Kerber 2003, 57). Moreover, hospitals in monopoly positions have only a slight appeal to render efficient services (Monopolkommission 2008, 317). Also, customers cannot chose which hospital is appropriate for them, if the hospitals are not in competition to others. As a result, customers have no other possibility than being treated in the monopoly hospital. Therefore, it is possible that the potential of quality improvement given through consolidations is not used completely (Monopolkommission 2008, 317). The quality competition in the health care system is the only guarantor of high-class care (Monopolkommission 2008, 318).
Furthermore, the access of competitors to the distributors can be hampered or becomes more expensive (Budzinski and Kerber 2003, 59). If hospitals build up a dominant position on the market by buying more hospitals, it comes to high administrative market access restrictions.

8

These can lead to allocation distortions which cannot be affected by the potential competition (Monopolkommission 2008, 318).

Greater market power can lead to higher prices for services in hospitals (Klauber, Robra and Schnellschmidt 2007, 60). A quality increasing effect of consolidations cannot be proven. On the one hand, it is obvious that there is a quality improvement because merged hospitals can use resources more efficiently. On the other hand, hospitals lose competitors and therewith the appeal to render high-class services. If there is only one hospital chain in an area, patients have to get treated there no matter how high the quality standards are. The patient has the free choice of hospitals concerning elective, planned treatments, however he mostly choses the nearest one (Monopolkommission 2008, 320). Another problem remains in the measurement of quality. Values of quality can be ascertained, for example the mortality and the cure rate, but these values not always give some indication of quality. Apart from the compliance of patients, many other factors have an influence on these values and it is not possible to regard quality isolated (Monopolkommission 2008, 320). However, empirical investigations show that there is a certain degree of transparency of quality in all the sectors controllable by patients. An increase of competitive pressure certainly leads to decreasing quality in not visible sectors (Monopolkommission 2008, 321).

Chapter 5
Conclusion

On the one hand, there is an allocative inefficiency because of the development of market power, but on the other hand, there is an economical increased efficiency because of the lower production costs. Now, it is important which element overbalances.

Another problem is that cost savings are not handed on to the customers or patients. Through the high market power, hospitals try to implement even higher prices. An increase of the treatment quality cannot be proven in this context, too. The higher the market concentration, the lower are the appeals for a quality improvement. Only a consolidation of smaller hospitals, which either specialise themselves or take over the standard care of a treatment area together, appears reasonable. They can save expenses because resources, like expensive equipment and staff, do not have to be available twice. With the aim to promote the quality competition, the monopoly commission recommends to develop a quality index (2008, 337) that shows treatment measures and cure rates of every single hospital. Patients could consult this register and chose a hospital for their treatment on the basis of the valuations.

It is believed that the overcapacity of hospital beds in German hospitals is going to rise from currently 6.5 per cent to more than 30 per cent in 2020 (Augurzky et al. 2009, 82) even though the number of patients in the stationary sector is going to increase by 3,8 per cent. Furthermore, it is assumed that the personnel requirements are going to increase by an average of 6 per cent. The personnel costs are steadily increasing, too (Augurzky et al. 2009, 14). Altogether, these developments lead to the closings of many hospitals because they are not in the economical position to bear cost increases (Augurzky et al. 2009, 14).

Especially for smaller hospitals, consolidations are an opportunity to persist. Through corporate use of resources, corporate purchase and a centralised management, great cost saving potentials can be used to increase the hospital's profitability (Steffen and Offermanns 2011, 7). A reduction of the range of services to one or two speciality departments can increase the profitability index (Augurzky et al. 2009, 15).

Hospitals, whose consolidations were successful, are deeply contented with the result and they would merge with other hospitals again (Steffen and Offermanns 2011, 7). If there is far-sighted scheduling and an early realisation of measures, costs can be saved and the profitability can be improved. A quality improving effect of consolidations has not been proven though.

Bibliography

Augurzky, Boris, Sebastian Krolop, Rosemarie Gülker, Christoph M. Schmidt, Hendrik Schmitz, Christoph Schwierz and Stefan Terkatz. 2009. *Krankenhaus Rating Report 2010: Licht und Schatten.* Essen: Rheinisch-Westfälisches Institut für Wirschaftsforschung.

Budzinski, Oliver and Wolfgang Kerber. 2003. *Megafusionen, Wettbewerb und Globalisierung. Praxis und Perspektiven der Wettbewerbspolitik.* Stuttgart: Lucius & Lucius Verlagsgesellschaft mbH.

Business Dictionary. 2011. *Consolidation.* http://www.businessdictionary.com/definition/consolidation.html (accessed 22 July 2011).

Monopolkommission. 2008. *Siebzehntes Hauptgutachten der Monopolkommission 2006/2007.* Ed. Deutscher Bundestag. Köln: Bundesanzeiger Verlagsgesellschaft mbH.

Eveslage, Karin. 2006. *Pflegediagnosen: praktisch und effizient.* Heidelberg: Springer Medizin Verlag.

Greulich, Andreas, Alberto Onetti, and Volker Schade. 2005. *Balanced Scorecard im Krankenhaus.* Heidelberg: Economica.

Köninger, Hubert. 2008. G-DRG und Kostenmanagement. In *DRG nach der Konvergenzphase*, ed. Bernhard Güntert and Günther Thiele, 99-122. Heidelberg: Economica.

Gesetz gegen Wettbewerbsbeschränkung. 2001. Beck.

Horzella, Andreas. 2010. *Wertsteigerung im M&A-Prozess: Erfolgsfaktoren – Instrumente – Kennzahlen.* Wiesbaden: Gabler.

Müller-Groh, Stefan G. 2002. Krankenhausfusionen: *Rechtsvergleich der Zusammenschlusskontrolle in Deutschland und den USA.* JD diss., University of Mannheim. http://madoc.bib.uni-mannheim.de/madoc/volltexte/2003/66/pdf/Dissertation-Mueller-Groh.pdf (accessed 22 July, 2011).

Urban, Dennis and Konrad Rippmann. 2007. Vorgehensweise und Erfolgsfaktoren bei Fusionsprozessen. In *Erfolgsfaktoren für marktorientiertes Fusionsmanagement in der Gesundheitswirtschaft*, ed. Wolfgang Hellmann, 11-18. Heidelberg: Economica.

Steffen, Petra and Offermanns, Matthias. 2011. *Erfolgskritische Faktoren von Krankenhausfusionen.* Düsseldorf: Deutsches Krankenhausinstitut.

Rippmann, Konrad. 2007. Unternehmensverbindungen in der Gesundheitswirtschaft – Treiber und Hindernisse. In *Erfolgsfaktoren für marktorientiertes Fusionsmanagement in der Gesundheitswirtschaft*, ed. Wolfgang Hellmann, 11-18. Heidelberg: Economica.

Vetter, Ulrich and Lutz Hoffmann. 2005. *Leistungsmanagement im Krankenhaus: G-DRGs.* Heidelberg: Springer Medizin Verlag.

Klauber, Jürgen, Bernt-Peter Robra and Henner Schnellschmidt. 2007. *Krankenhaus-Report 2006: Schwerpunkt: Krankenhausmarkt im Umbruch.* Stuttgart: Schattauer GmbH.